Carpal Tunnel Syndrome & Overuse Injuries

Carpal Tunnel Syndrome & Overuse Injuries

Prevention, Treatment & Recovery

Tammy Crouch
Michael Madden, D.C.

North Atlantic Books
Berkeley, California

Carpal Tunnel Syndrome and Overuse Injuries:
Prevention, Treatment, and Recovery

ISBN 1-55643-135-X

Published by
North Atlantic Books
P.O. Box 12327
Berkeley, California 94701–9998

Cover photograph by Richard Blair
Cover and book design by Paula Morrison

Printed in the United States of America by Malloy Lithographing

Carpal Tunnel Syndrome and Overuse Injuries: Prevention, Treatment, and Recovery is sponsored by the Society for the Study of Native Arts and Sciences, a nonprofit educational corporation whose goals are to develop an educational and crosscultural perspective linking various scientific, social, and artistic fields; to nurture a holistic view of arts, sciences, humanities, and healing; and to publish and distribute literature on the relationship of mind, body, and nature.

To John and Erin

ACKNOWLEDGEMENTS

The authors would like to thank everyone who offered suggestions, information, personal experiences, advice, and support during this project, particularly Dr. Dena Lendrum, David Esposito, Colleen Timmons L.Ac., Dr. William Previte, Dr. Robert Gelb, Dr. John Ford, Greg Bilg, William Mann L.Ac., Dr. Tom Humphries, Lisa Williams, Renea Wagner, Liz Mendoza, Sharon Allen, Linda Hardin and the staff at Madden Chiropractic Clinic, Dr. Stuart Marshall and Dr. David Haaland, and everyone else who gave us so much encouragement along the way.

Thanks to Cheance Adair for the illustrations in Chapters 7 and 8, and for your generous help throughout the entire project.

Last, a special thank you to John Crouch for support and assistance far above and beyond the call of duty.

Models for photographs and illustrations are Tracy Kuerbis, Renea Wagner, John Crouch, Dr. Michael Sullivan, Liz Mendoza, Dr. Dena Lendrum, Lalyn Bellman, Cheance Adair and Rob Balaam. Authors' photograph by Expressly Portraits.

TABLE OF CONTENTS

TABLE OF CONTENTS

TABLE OF CONTENTS

INTRODUCTION

At one time or another, everyone has had the sensation of "pins and needles" or a hand or arm "falling asleep" or aching. Usually, just shaking or rubbing the affected limb is enough to bring the feeling back. But for the tens of millions of people with the condition known as Carpal Tunnel Syndrome (CTS), the feeling doesn't come back quite so easily, if at all.

During the past few years there has been a dramatic increase in the number of CTS cases. The majority of people diagnosed with CTS are involved with some kind of repetitive task in the workplace or home involving the use of hands or fingers. Application of force, pressure from hard work surfaces, vibration, and certain hand tools have all been shown to increase the incidence of CTS. Repeated pressure in the joint as well as the increased size of muscles and tendons pressing on the median nerve in the wrist all serve to exacerbate the problem.

Who gets it?

- computer operators
- retail clerks
- waiters/waitresses
- assembly workers
- musicians
- hairstylists
- typists
- sign language interpreters
- construction workers
- butchers

Our reasons for writing this book are many. We shared an increasing sense of alarm at the numbers of Carpal Tunnel Syndrome cases, and frustration in the knowledge that these injuries can be prevented in most cases.

Tammy Crouch: Eight years ago I began noticing numbness and tingling in my right hand. I had worked as a Sign Language Interpreter for four years, and enjoyed my job. When my family doctor diagnosed Carpal Tunnel Syndrome, I didn't make the connection between the hours of repetitive movement I performed daily and the increasing weakness and loss of feeling in what was soon to be both of my hands. Surgery was recommended, and was very successful. Unfortunately, I went right back into a non-stop work routine, and within a year had Carpal Tunnel Syndrome a second time. Having a second surgery (this time on my elbow to relieve ulnar neuritis) opened my eyes to what the repetitive movement required by my job was doing to me. After being told by my orthopedic surgeon that there wasn't much hope for regaining the full use of my arm and hand, I decided to become educated about these injuries—not only for myself but for the 90% of my coworkers who were by now experiencing problems, too. I began working closely with other interpreters and students on prevention and recovery, and we saw a gradual decline in the number of injuries. Whether you find relief from acupuncture, chiropractic, or traditional medicine, this book will give you the information you need to make responsible, informed choices. I was able to recover from this potentially disabling condition, and with a few changes in work and personal habits most sufferers of overuse injuries can do the same.

Dr. Michael Madden: In the last five or six years, in my private practice, I have begun to see an alarmingly higher incidence of Carpal Tunnel Syndrome. It is a problem that affects people both personally and professionally. Once the condition has gotten to a point that it is significantly interfering with a person's life, it is oftentimes very difficult to completely fix. In my office, the overwhelming majority of people who have it have been those who perform repetitive actions in their work or private lives. The purpose of this book is to help outline the different types of treatments for this syndrome, and even more so, to identify as early as possible the presence of symptoms and list ways of preventing them.

1

WHAT IS CARPAL TUNNEL SYNDROME?

The condition known as Carpal Tunnel Syndrome, Cumulative Trauma Disorder, Repetitive Motion Injury, or Occupational Neuritis was described as long ago as 1854 by Sir James Paget as chronic compression of the **median nerve**. In 1947 Dr. George Phalen made his first diagnosis of Carpal Tunnel Syndrome, and since then this debilitating injury has been the subject of extensive research and attention from all facets of the medical community. It is estimated that at least 10% of all workers performing duties requiring prolonged or repetitive movement of the hands will be affected by Carpal Tunnel Syndrome.

This book will explore a variety of ways to prevent overuse injuries and alleviate symptoms, but first let's get an understanding of the anatomy of the hand and wrist.

THE CARPAL TUNNEL

The **carpal tunnel** is a narrow opening in the palm side of the wrist made up of eight wrist (or **carpal**) bones [Figure 1]. Three walls of the tunnel are made up of these carpal bones, while the fourth is formed by the tough transverse carpal ligament. Through the tunnel pass nine **tendons**, tough bands of connective tissue

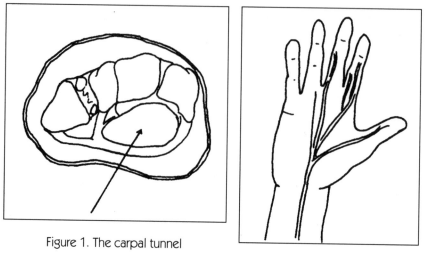

Figure 1. The carpal tunnel

Figure 2. The median nerve

that attach the muscles of the arm to the bones in the hand. These tendons are the four profundus tendons, four superficialis tendons, and the flexor pollicis longus tendon. Also passing through the carpal tunnel is the **median nerve**, the nerve that carries signals between the hand and the brain [Fig. 2]. The median nerve performs two functions: **sensory**—it allows the hand to feel sensations, and **motor**—it allows the hand to move and do things.

CARPAL TUNNEL SYNDROME

Many factors can cause pressure on the median nerve. If for any reason the contents of the carpal tunnel become larger or swollen, or the tunnel itself becomes smaller, the median nerve can become pinched or irritated. Inflammation and swelling of the nerve generally lead to a variety of symptoms which are collectively called **Carpal Tunnel Syndrome**. These sensory and motor symptoms include:

Sensory	Motor
numbness, especially at night	loss of hand strength
tingling	weakness of thumb
burning	smaller thumb muscles
coldness	clumsiness
stiff, swollen joints	aching

These symptoms can be felt in the hand (especially the thumb, index, and middle fingers), wrist, up into the elbow and even in the shoulder. Often these feelings are worse at night, and the pain and tingling can be severe enough to wake a person from a sound sleep. In the early stages, relief can be obtained by shaking the hand out or massaging the area. Consistent use of the hand will gradually increase the symptoms in most cases, and as the problem becomes worse, the motor portion of the nerve is involved. It becomes more difficult to perform small, specific tasks such as buttoning clothes, picking things up, etc., and hand strength is often affected.

"It's like a feeling of pins and needles."

"Feels as if my hand is asleep."

"I have shooting pains down my forearm."

"My handwriting became illegible."

"Feels like I just hit my 'funny bone.'"

"I began dropping things . . . my grip became weak."

"Both hands and wrists became swollen."

"At night my hands would fall asleep from wrist to fingertips and **ache**!"

Why do my symptoms seem worse at night?

Blood flows through your system much slower at night, which can enlarge the blood vessels at the carpal tunnel. The increased amount of blood puts pressure on the nerve. This explains the increased numbness, tingling, and pain some people experience at night.

Also, the position of your hands and arms as you sleep can play a major part in worsening symptoms of CTS. If you sleep with your hands in a hyperflexed or hyperextended position you may very well wake up with hands that feel as if they are "asleep." Changing habits that occur while you sleep is difficult, but it can be done. Many CTS patients find that wearing wrist splints to bed keep the hands in a more neutral position and relieve some of the pressure on the median nerve.

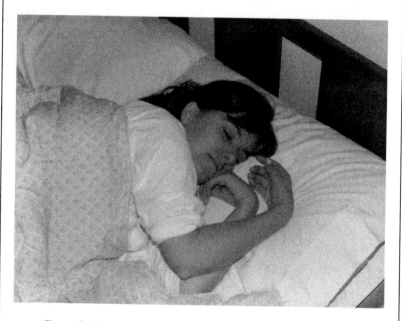

Figure 3. Sleeping positions like this can worsen symptoms.

ACCUMULATIVE TRAUMA

Carpal Tunnel Syndrome can be caused by a variety of factors, from an injury to the wrist area to a problem with general health. This book will focus on Carpal Tunnel Syndrome caused by **accumulative trauma**.

When the hand is used repeatedly over long periods of time in an awkward position, especially with excessive amounts of **hyperflexion** and/or **hyperextension** [see Figures 4 and 5], the joints and tendons can become inflamed and swollen, compressing the median nerve. That pressure can lead to changes in the sensory and motor aspects of the hand.

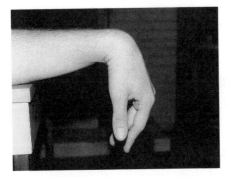

Figure 4. Hyperflexion

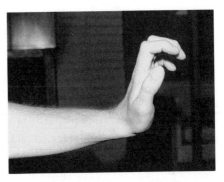

Figure 5. Hyperextension

OTHER CAUSES OF CTS

There are other causes of Carpal Tunnel Syndrome that should be ruled out by your physician before you attempt the self-help measures described in this book. These include systemic conditions that relate to the whole body, such as:

Diabetes Mellitis	Kidney Dialysis
Hypothyroidism	Oral Contraceptives
Pregnancy	Menopause

Or conditions that affect the actual narrowing of the carpal tunnel, like:

Pagets Bone Disease   Multiple Myeloma
Acromegaly   Pisiform Hamate Syndrome
Improperly set fractures or dislocations
Rheumatoid, Osteo and Gouty Arthritis

• Again, if you are experiencing any of the symptoms of Carpal Tunnel Syndrome, please see your doctor without delay to be sure you are not suffering from any of the above conditions.

RELATED DISORDERS

Carpal Tunnel Syndrome is not the only injury related to overuse of the hands and arms. The forearm, elbow, and shoulder are also subject to wear and tear from overuse, and there are some specific problems that affect them as well. These other disorders include:

Ulnar nerve irritation: Generally, compression of the ulnar nerve (what people often refer to as the "funny bone"—see Fig. 6) at the inside of the elbow. Repetitive trauma can lead to a thickening in this region, usually due to a buildup of scar tissue. The patient feels a tingling sensation in the hand, inability to separate the fingers and altered sensation of the fourth and fifth fingers.

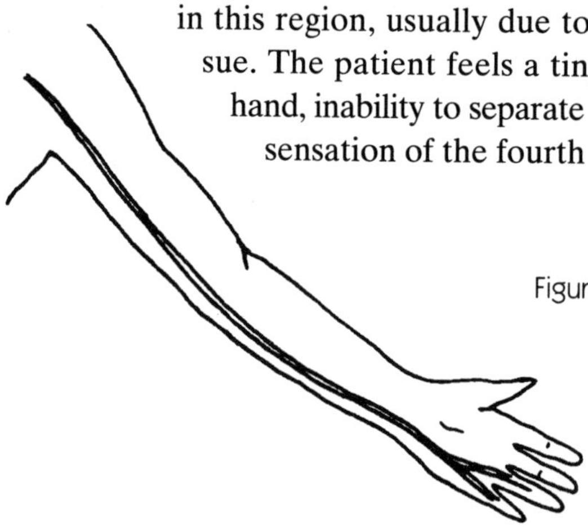

Figure 6. Ulnar nerve

Tendonitis: Inflammation of the tendon at the medial or outer edge of the elbow [Fig. 7]. Injury occurs when the elbow is extended repeatedly, often combined with twisting or flexing the elbow and arm, especially against resistance.

The result is considerable contraction of the extensor supinator muscles of the forearm. More common than ulnar nerve injury, tendonitis is often called "tennis elbow" or "golfer's elbow." There is often a feeling of pain that can spread down the en-

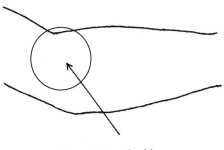

Figure 7. Tendonitis

tire length of the forearm as well as up into the shoulder. Grip and general forearm strength are usually affected.

Tenosynovitis: Also known as **DeQuervain's Disease**, tenosynovitis affects a small tunnel along the thumb side of the wrist that transports some extensor and thumb tendons [Fig. 8]. In this disease, there is inflammation which narrows the lining of the tunnel, resulting in pain and tenderness around the affected wrist and thumb.

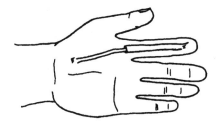

Figure 8. Site of tenosynovitis

7

Now you have an idea of what Carpal Tunnel Syndrome is and what it isn't. Only a trained professional can tell you if what you are experiencing is, in fact, Carpal Tunnel Syndrome. The next chapter will help you get an understanding of the kinds of health care that are available to you.

2

GETTING HELP

Now, assuming you have ruled out all other potential causes for your tingling, painful hands, what is the next step? What do health professionals do when presented with a case like yours? In this chapter we will describe a variety of theories and practices to help you make the most informed choice about your treatment.

TRADITIONAL AND NONTRADITIONAL MEDICINE

Most of us are familiar with the practice of traditional Western medicine—the diagnosis and treatment of disease and maintenance of health by a licensed medical doctor, using medication and/or surgery. The first doctor you see about your symptoms may be your family doctor, who may or may not be familiar with overuse injuries. Chapter 10 gives you some specific questions to ask when choosing a physician to treat your case, and in the Appendix you will find an "Overuse Injury Checklist" to help you keep track of your symptoms and provide specific information to help your physician make a diagnosis.

If you are interested in seeing a medical doctor, you may consider visiting a specialist. Orthopedic surgeons who specialize in hand disorders are familiar with Carpal Tunnel Syndrome as well as other overuse injuries affecting the arms. You should expect to be thoroughly examined, using some of the diagnostic techniques listed in Chapter 3.

The physician should ask not only about your symptoms, but also about your activities, lifestyle, medical history, and emotional and physical stresses—factors that help determine both how you got the injury as well as what you need to do to get better.

Medical doctors who specialize in sports medicine are usually also experienced in treating CTS, and work closely with physical therapists in rehabilitating the injured limb. A good treatment plan will not only help repair the injury but also help you strengthen the arms and the entire upper body to prevent the condition from recurring.

"ALTERNATIVE" MEDICINE

There are also less traditional methods of treatment that may not be as familiar to you, but have proven successful in treating CTS. Each person is different; what worked for the injured cashier at the grocery store may be all wrong for your particular case. It can take some effort to find the best treatment for you.

Whether you call it alternative, holistic, or natural medicine, there are numerous health practitioners who employ techniques other than drug therapy and surgery to help their patients get well. And rather than seeing the choice between orthodox and nontraditional medicine as an "either/or" situation, different healing professions *can* work together, complementing each other. The idea of mixing traditional Western medicine with the more "holistic" approaches of, say, acupuncture, homeopathy, or chiropractic, is a new one. But it may be the most effective way to successfully serve *all* of a patient's needs in the treatment of injury or disease. There are times when medicine or surgery are not enough, and supplemental care in a less traditional mode will turn the case around. Likewise, an acupuncturist may refer a client out for surgery when an injured nerve isn't responding to treatment. Finding a physician or therapist with an open mind and the awareness of the ways in which various specialties can enhance rather than compete with each other is a powerful first step toward recovery from injury.

CHIROPRACTIC

Chiropractic is the largest natural healing profession in the United States (47,000 practitioners). Chiropractors believe that many musculoskeletal problems are caused by different types of pressure on the nervous system, and that the loss of normal nerve activity can also lead to disorders of certain organic systems. Carpal Tunnel Syndrome involves the nerves of the wrist, but those nerves connect all the way up through the arm, shoulder, and neck. If there is pressure on a nerve in the spine, the effects can reach all the way down to the fingertips.

A chiropractic physician will restore the nervous system to normal by "adjusting" the patient—relieving pressure by manipulating a particular joint which is **fixated**, or "stuck," back in the proper direction, thus enabling the nervous system to heal or regulate itself.

There are generally two schools of thought related to chiropractic care. Some chiropractors limit their treatment to manipulation of the spine. On the other side are those who employ a variety of techniques in addition to manipulation: massage, electrical therapy like ultrasound and interferential, nutrition, homeopathy.

Subluxations (misalignments of the spine) or fixations in the wrist, elbow, shoulder, or neck can interfere with the nerves in that area. Problems originating above the wrist can affect the nerves going to the wrist. Cervical spine (neck) problems especially are often noted with Carpal Tunnel Syndrome. Medical studies refer to this as the "double crush phenomenon." When a nerve is compressed in one area (the neck, for example) it then becomes more susceptible to further damage elsewhere (Osterman, A.: Causes of Failure in Carpal Tunnel Surgery. 53rd Annual Meeting of the American Academy of Orthopedic Surgeons, 1986).

What is ultrasound?

Ultrasound uses high frequency sound waves to increase blood flow to an injured area, warm muscles, and relieve pain. Ultrasound can also reduce tissue inflammation and edema (swelling). More effective than simple vibration or heat, ultrasound penetrates deep into the muscles and joints. Combined with other therapies (physical therapy, chiropractic), ultrasound can effectively relieve symptoms of CTS when administered by a trained professional.

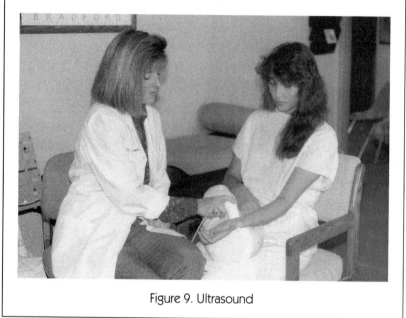

Figure 9. Ultrasound

Adjusting the vertebrae in the spine relieves the primary compression, then the arm and wrist can be treated to improve function and reduce symptoms. Medical research has shown that the chance of a successful outcome from CTS surgery is greatly reduced if there is also a problem in the neck that is left untreated, so chiropractic physicians believe it is vital to look beyond the wrist when treating CTS.

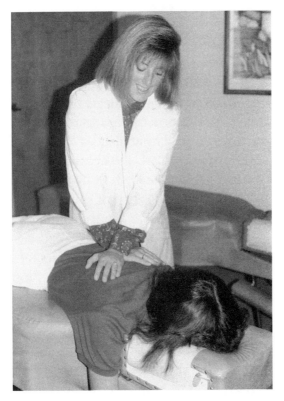

Figure 10. Chiropractic

Some Doctors of Chiropractic use their hands to perform an adjustment, while others use instruments. Most rely on orthodox methods of diagnosis, such as the use of X-rays, orthopedic and neurological tests, and may use physical therapy, including massage and ultrasound, when indicated. A visit to the chiropractor is pleasant for most patients. And though the "cracking" sound you hear while being adjusted manually by a chiropractor can be unnerving at first, there is often a feeling of relief and "loosening up" afterward. Medicare, Worker's Compensation, and most private insurance companies will cover the cost of chiropractic treatment. Your chiropractor may also work with you on diet, exercise, and lifestyle, with the idea that overall health greatly affects the process of recovery from injury.

OSTEOPATHY

Osteopaths support the idea, as do chiropractors, that achieving a structural balance will bring about healing. Osteopathic physicians (D.O.'s) undergo a traditional medical education, which is then followed by additional coursework emphasizing the muscular and skeletal systems. Like chiropractors, osteopaths use manipulation of the spine to correct injuries or imbalances within the neuro-muscular-skeletal system, but they are also licensed to prescribe medication or perform surgery if needed. In that respect, osteopathic physicians are in the unique position of being able to help the body to heal itself through the use of hands-on manipulative therapy, along with the ability to offer treatment with drugs or surgery if necessary. Osteopaths may also emphasize the importance of exercises and stretches to increase range of motion, thus restoring the full functioning of the blood and lymphatic systems.

ACUPUNCTURE

One of the oldest known systems of medicine in the world, acupuncture has been practiced for at least 5,000 years. Acupuncture involves the insertion of very fine needles into specific points on the body. It is believed that acupuncture restores the balance of **chi**—the energy that makes up each being's life force. Chi flows throughout the body along pathways called **meridians**, and illness occurs when the pathways become blocked. Practitioners of traditional Chinese medicine seek to release this trapped energy and restore the body to health.

In acupuncture therapy, specific points are stimulated to restore balance to the body. Again, with Carpal Tunnel Syndrome treatment is *not* necessarily confined to the hands, wrists, and arms. Treating the neck, back, and shoulders as well will begin to heal the entire length of the injured nerve. Acupuncturists may also use transcutaneous nerve stimulation (TENS), heat treatments,

TENS

A small, battery-operated device, wired to electrode patches attached to the patient's skin, the TENS (transcutaneous electrical nerve stimulation) unit is gaining in popularity as an effective pain reliever for all kinds of symptoms. Like acupuncture, the electrical pulses seem to stimulate the body's own natural painkillers. The patient generally feels nothing more than a mild tingling. Ask your doctor or physical therapist if TENS is an option for you.

and herbs, not only to heal the injury and relieve symptoms, but to bring about balance to the entire system. The philosophy of Oriental medicine supports the idea that a healthy, balanced system is less prone to injury and disease.

Acupuncture stimulates the release of **endorphins**, the body's own natural pain reliever, from the brain. Does acupuncture hurt? Depends on who you ask. Most patients feel comfortable throughout the treatment—the needles used are extremely fine and generally insertion is painless. A few people report a feeling of mild discomfort as the needle is put into place, but this is usually very brief and followed almost immediately by a feeling of calm and relaxation as the treatment proceeds. The needles may be gently twisted while in place, or heat or a mild electrical current may be applied.

Acupuncture is used to relieve a wide variety of problems from headaches to premenstrual syndrome, even as an anesthetic during surgery. And although its acceptance in the Western world has been slow, many insurance companies will now cover the cost of acupuncture. Acupuncturists are also interested in treating the total person; you will be carefully examined and have an extensive history taken at your first visit. In addition to treatment with needles, you may be given herbs or homeopathic remedies (see Homeopathy). Your pulse may be checked at several points throughout your body, and your skin, nails, and even tongue examined in order for the acupuncturist to get a sense of the state of your general health.

PHYSICAL THERAPY

Physical therapists assist in rehabilitation and restoration of normal bodily function after illness or injury through the use of therapeutic exercises, hydro[water]therapy, and the application of various forms of energy: electrotherapy, ultrasound, and interferential current therapy.

A physical therapist can also teach you about proper work habits, posture, and how you can achieve a more healthy lifestyle. Chiropractors and medical doctors sometimes work with physical therapists when treating CTS and overuse injuries, and most patients find the experience pleasant and helpful.

Most states require a referral from your doctor allowing you to be treated by a physical therapist.

Interferential Current Therapy

A type of electrical treatment, interferential current therapy has become quite popular in recent years in the treatment of Carpal Tunnel Syndrome and other overuse injuries. The medium-frequency current penetrates deep into the joint or muscle, to increase circulation—reducing edema, swelling, and inflammation, stimulating the release of pain-reducing hormones in the body, and increasing overall muscle tone. A session with the interferential unit lasts about 10–15 minutes in most cases, and the feeling of the electrical pulse is somewhat odd but not uncomfortable. Results can be dramatic, and longer lasting than treatment with ultrasound.

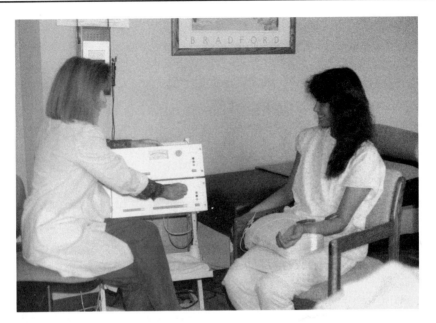

Figure 11. Interferential Current Therapy

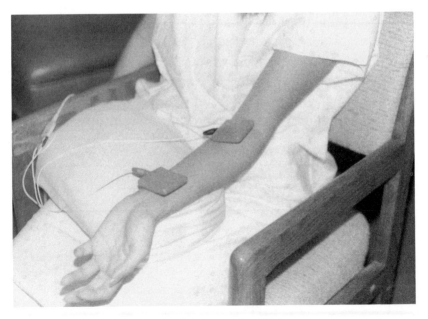

Figure 12. Pads in place for CTS therapy

MASSAGE

Massage involves stroking and kneading the body to loosen the muscle tissues, increase movement of joints and removal of toxins, and restore the flow of energy. Massage increases blood flow to the muscles, and can aid in reducing the stiffness and swelling that often accompany injury. A massage therapist familiar with overuse-type injuries can work wonders in relieving pain and numbness. Don't be afraid to shop around until you find a therapist with the right touch. There are many types of massage, some gentle, some deep. Swedish, Shiatsu, Trager, Esalen . . . you may hear lots of exotic-sounding terms for the various techniques used by massage therapists. The type of massage you receive will depend on the therapist's training, background, and personal philosophy. Most massage therapists are an excellent source of information and guidance on injury prevention and home care. And because they, too, work with their hands and arms quite a bit, they often have firsthand knowledge about overuse injuries.

The massage therapist should be experienced enough to be able to adjust his/her technique to your particular needs, and explain what s/he is doing and why. Often CTS patients find they enjoy a deep massage to help work out the "knots" in their necks and shoulders; however, a gentle approach feels best if you have lots of inflammation, when deep work can actually do more harm than good. Find the technique that works best for you.

HOMEOPATHY

Homeopathic medicine is based on one simple principle: "like cures like." The homeopath considers the whole person when presented with a set of symptoms. Not only the physical but also the patient's emotional and mental processes are considered when making a diagnosis. A remedy is chosen which closely fits all aspects of your symptoms and will stimulate your body to heal itself. The correct remedy is one which produces reactions similar to those the patient is experiencing, activating and strengthening the patient's own system in response to the remedy.

Homeopathic remedies are made from natural substances (flowers, minerals, roots, and oils, for example) which are sequentially diluted. The more a substance is diluted, the higher its potency. In other words, according to homeopaths, a minute dose of the correct substance will activate the patient's own defenses to attack the illness. Homeopaths may also make recommendations about diet, lifestyle, or exercise to help you bring your life into balance. Homeopathy can work well in conjunction with most other therapies, even traditional Western medicine. Homeopathic remedies may be taken orally in the form of pills or liquid, or applied topically in ointments and creams. An excellent homeopathic cream for topical application to injured arms and hands is called **Traumeel** (check your local natural food store or see Appendix C for ordering information).

As you can see, there are many choices in health care available for people with Carpal Tunnel Syndrome. It's just a matter of finding the particular method and practitioner that works best for you.

3

MAKING
THE DIAGNOSIS

Regardless of the type of health-care practitioner you choose, your examination should include *at least* one of the following diagnostic tests to determine conclusively whether or not what you are experiencing is Carpal Tunnel Syndrome.

ORTHOPEDIC TESTING

The two most common tests done to determine problems with the median nerve are the wrist flexion test, or **Phalen's test**, and the median nerve percussion test, or **Tinel's test**.

The wrist flexion test is done by placing the back of the hands together in a bent position, completely flexed, but without force [Fig. 13]. If there is any numbness, tingling or pain within sixty seconds, the test is positive.

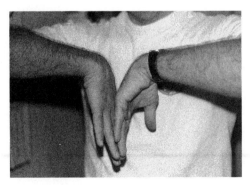

Figure 13. Phalen's test

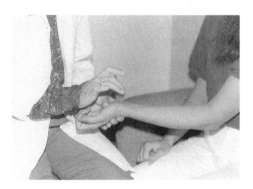

Tinel's test is performed by tapping the area over the median nerve on the palm side of the hand [Fig. 14]. Again, if tingling or numbness is felt, the test is positive.

Figure 14. Tinel's test

Another test used to determine sensitivity in the area is the **Semmes-Weinstein test** [Fig. 15], where a variety of sizes and weights of plastic rods are touched against the fingertips to test

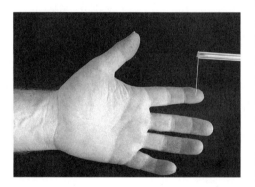

the degree of sensitivity compared to the normal level. This test can sometimes reveal Carpal Tunnel Syndrome symptoms before they become serious, or even before they are noticed.

Figure 15. Semmes-Weinstein test

The **Vibrometer test** also determines levels of sensitivity through the use of vibration against the fingers. Deviations from

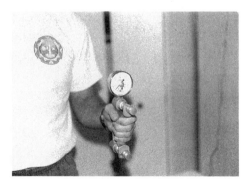

the norm can sometimes be present even when the patient has not yet experienced any symptoms.

An instrument called a **Dynamometer** is used to measure the strength of

Figure 16. Dynamometer testing

the patient's grip. The patient squeezes the Dynamometer [Fig. 16] and the readings are recorded. The dominant hand (usually the one you write with) is generally 5–10 lbs. stronger than the nondominant hand. Differences from that norm can indicate hand, arm, or even neck involvement.

APPLIED KINESIOLOGY

Some health-care practitioners employ a method of muscle testing to discover weaknesses or other muscular problems. Created by chiropractor Dr. George Goodheart, Applied Kinesiology combines theories of acupuncture and manipulation to measure neurological functioning throughout the body.

X-RAYS, COMPUTERIZED TOMOGRAPHY, AND MAGNETIC RESONANCE IMAGING

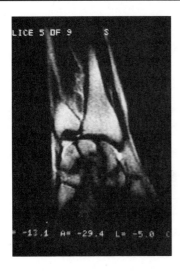

Figure 17. MRI of a Hand

X-rays of the wrist and arm may be recommended by an M.D., chiropractor, or osteopath. If abnormalities occur, two tests which show a three-dimensional view of the area and the actual size of the tunnel can be helpful. These are the **CT scan** (also called **CAT scan** or **Computerized Tomography**) or the **MRI (Magnetic Resonance Imaging)**. The two tests are similar, but the MRI [Fig. 17] uses principles of magnetism, rather than X-rays like the CT scan, to view the contents of the carpal tunnel. These tests are not only valuable

23

in diagnosing Carpal Tunnel Syndrome, but can be used after treatment to determine progress and response to treatment.

EMG—ELECTROMYOGRAPHY

The test that generally defines the "official" presence of Carpal Tunnel Syndrome is **electromyography**, or **EMG**, a nerve conduction test generally performed by a **neurologist** (a medical doctor who specializes in nerve disorders). The EMG shows any alteration in the way the nerves and muscles work. During the test, nerves and muscles in various areas undergo electrical stimulation, then are observed for abnormal electrical activity when at rest, upon insertion of a small needle, and during contraction (making a fist, for example).

Wave patterns can indicate nerve damage, muscle weakness, and specific muscle diseases, such as myasthenia gravis. Electromyography can be uncomfortable for the patient, particularly when the needles are inserted. However, with an accuracy rate of 90%, it is a very reliable test to indicate any problems with the median nerve.

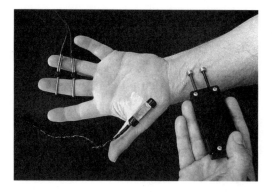

Figure 18. EMG Testing

4

STAGE
I

The type of treatment your doctor or therapist recommends will depend on several factors: his/her particular philosophy, your work or personal habits that affect your injury, and the severity of your symptoms. We have divided the stages of CTS into three categories: **Stage I**, mild symptoms with negative test results; **Stage II**, moderate symptoms with positive results from orthopedic and/or neurological testing; and **Stage III**, moderate to severe symptoms with significant abnormalities on the electromyographic studies. Chapters 4, 5, and 6 discuss symptoms as well as some ideas for treatment for each stage.

STAGE I

At this early stage, symptoms are mild and tests for damage to the nerve are negative. You may be feeling some intermittent numbness or tingling, and perhaps pain in the wrist or forearm. Usually, a short rest period, a massage, or a session with the chiropractor, physical therapist, or acupuncturist bring relief that lasts for weeks. With a few changes in work habits and lifestyle, chances for a complete recovery are excellent. Recommendations for treatment will certainly vary from doctor to doctor; however, we found the following to be the most common suggestions given to CTS patients in Stage I:

• **Rest.** Nearly every practitioner we asked, regardless of specialty, recommended rest from aggravating activities and modification of daily habits to allow the injured nerve to heal. Regular breaks during any activity involving the hands and arms is often enough to halt the problem before it worsens. It's as simple as taking a break. Be aware of your own physical limitations when performing any task requiring repetitive movement. Are you becoming fatigued or stiffening up? Have your hands or neck been in an awkward position for a prolonged period of time? Most people need to take a short break after every 20–40 minutes of continuous activity to stretch, walk around, or just relax the hands and arms.

• **Immobilization** through the use of **wrist splints**, which hold the wrist in a nonflexed position [Fig. 19]. The splint should fit well but not so tight that circulation is impaired. A too-tight splint can do more harm than good. It should *limit* range of movement, but not prevent it entirely. You should be able to move the wrist slightly (about 10% of your normal range of motion) while wear-

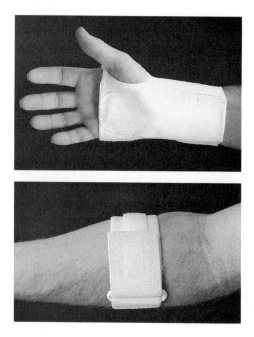

ing the splint. Splints are highly effective for many people, especially when worn at night, and in many cases they can be worn *while* performing tasks that aggravate your symptoms.

Figure 19. Wrist splint

• A **forearm brace** is effective in relieving pain in the elbow and forearm. These simple bands are often used for "tennis el-

Figure 20. Forearm brace

bow," and can be purchased in most drug or medical supply stores for around $5.00. As with the wrist splint, do not tighten the forearm brace so much that you cut off circulation to your hand. It should fit snugly but comfortably.

• The use of **ice packs** can help to reduce inflammation. Apply the pack to the affected areas, right on the hand, wrist or elbow if needed, throughout the day for 10–15 minute periods. You can even massage the injured area with the ice pack for extra relief. If the coldness hurts your skin, try wrapping the pack in a towel. If discomfort persists, discontinue using the ice pack. (Don't have an ice pack? A bag of frozen peas or corn works just as well in an emergency.)

• The application of **moist heat**, particularly to the neck and shoulder areas, can help to relax tight muscles. Wet a towel with hot water (*comfortably* hot—don't burn yourself), wring it out well, wrap it around a hot water bottle and lie down on your back so that your neck and shoulders are resting on the towel. Relax for 10–15 minutes. A regular heating pad can feel good as well, but moist heat is more penetrating and its effects are longer lasting. There are now special moist heat pads that are easy to use and can be purchased for around $10.00; check your local pharmacy.

ICE vs. HEAT

When should you apply heat to an injury, and when is ice the best choice? Ice is used when there is inflammation to prevent or reduce swelling, particularly in the acute stages. The application of cold constricts blood vessels in the area and prevents them from bleeding. Heat *draws* blood to an injured area and the increased circulation assists in the body's attempts to heal itself. Heat works best after the acute stage has passed, rather than immediately after an injury or when inflammation is present, when it could actually worsen swelling.

• **Anti-inflammatory medications**, such as aspirin, ibuprofen (like Motrin or Advil), or a prescription medication to reduce inflammation are often prescribed by medical doctors to ease pain and numbness. These drugs *can* effectively relieve symptoms (aspirin and ibuprofen both inhibit the body's production of prostaglandins, a substance that triggers pain), but prolonged use may do more harm than good. Gastrointestinal disturbances, stomach bleeding, and headaches are a few of the known side effects of aspirin and ibuprofen. Prescription muscle relaxants or narcotic pain relievers can cause dizziness, nausea, and some are dangerously addictive. Be sure to ask your physician about any medication s/he recommends, and even if symptoms subside considerably, it is still important for you to make changes in the habits that caused the injury in the first place. Medication can be extremely helpful in alleviating the initial symptoms, but should not be seen as a "cure" for an injury caused by overuse.

What about acetaminophen?

Marketed under brand names like Datril and Tylenol, acetaminophen is an effective pain reliever, but does not reduce inflammation like aspirin or ibuprofen.

• **Massage** is extremely effective in relaxing tight and sometimes spasmed muscles in the arm, shoulders, neck, and middle back. When there is no massage therapist around, an electric massager can help to relax sore, tight muscles, as well, and can allow you to work on hard-to-reach areas like the upper back. We've heard of offices with a high rate of overuse injuries (data entry operators, for example) who began keeping an electric massager or two in a convenient place in the office for workers to use during break times. One of the best is Conair's Sonassage Sonic Pain Reliever, which comes with a variety of attachments, including one specially designed for the hand and fingers. (See Appendix C for ordering information.)

• **Home treatment** to insure maximum neck mobility. If your neck has certain structural problems that affect your injury, cervical exercises [see Chapter 7], home traction devices (you'll need a doctor's recommendation for this), and cervical pillows can all help you maintain your health on a daily basis. Remember to first have a physician check for hereditary bone abnormalities, osteo-arthritis, and muscle, ligament, or disc damage from accidents.

• Care for any underlying systemic disease. If your general health is poor or your symptoms are worsened by any of the conditions we discussed in Chapter 1, begin taking care of yourself *now.* See a physician for a treatment plan designed for your particular needs.

In the mild stage, damage to the nerve is still limited and more serious problems *can* be avoided. It is important to remember that the injury is seldom confined to the wrist and hand area; in accumulated injuries the entire arm, shoulder and even neck are often involved, and for maximum effectiveness treatment should also be directed to these areas. There may also be pain around the elbow, and the shoulders, middle back, and neck are generally stiff, tight, and sore.

5

STAGE
II

In **Stage II** Carpal Tunnel Syndrome, symptoms are moderate, and orthopedic and neurological tests are *positive*. The previous methods we've discussed should still be continued at this stage; they may bring a great deal of relief and prevent the injury from worsening. When diagnostic tests, particularly the neurological tests, are positive, there is damage to the nerve requiring a somewhat more aggressive approach. Taking a ten-minute break may not be enough any more. Patients with Stage II CTS often report that symptoms like pain and tingling continue for some time even after the aggravating activity is stopped. It takes a longer massage, extended periods wearing a splint or forearm brace, or more frequent visits to the doctor for therapy to obtain relief.

The following are some additional ideas you can try on your own at home, in any stage of CTS:

• **Diet and nutrition**: studies have shown that in some cases a deficiency of vitamin B_6 may play a role in the development of Carpal Tunnel Syndrome. 100 mg. per day of B_6 improved symptoms considerably for many patients. B_6 is also a natural diuretic, relieving water retention which can worsen symptoms. (Water retention can explain the increased pain and tingling some women experience premenstrually and during pregnancy.) B_6 supplements should be taken with care; ironically, excessive amounts can cause the very symptoms you are trying to relieve. Birth control pills can deplete the body's supply of B_6, so if you are on the pill and experiencing symptoms of CTS, consider supplementing your diet with B_6.

Another factor to consider is sugar; high levels of refined sugar in the diet have been shown to reduce the body's overall ability to fight off inflammations, colds, allergies, etc. Avoid sugar completely when inflammation is present, and reduce your regular intake on a daily basis. Get into the habit of reaching for a piece of fruit instead of a doughnut or a candy bar. You may notice a big difference not only in your hands and arms, but in your energy level, moods, and immune system.

• **Topical application** of homeopathic remedies, ginger soaks /compresses, or salves like tiger balm or Mineral Ice® provide temporary relief.

Ginger compress

Grate fresh ginger and wrap in a cloth. Squeeze the cloth so the juice drips down into a pot of hot water, then dip a hand towel into the ginger water. Wring out, then apply hot (but not scalding) to the injured area. Cover with a dry towel to retain heat. Replace every 3–5 minutes.

• **Paraffin Bath:** A paraffin bath is a warm mixture of paraffin wax and mineral oil (four parts wax to one part oil). The wax and oil are melted down, and the hand is dipped repeatedly into the mixture, building up layers of paraffin. The heat deeply penetrates into the muscles and tendons, and has been found to help with arthritic pain and stiffness. Wrap the paraffin-coated hand in a warm, moist towel and allow the heat to penetrate the hand for 15–20 minutes. Then peel away the wax, and massage and gently stretch and exercise the hand. You can melt the wax yourself (carefully!) on the stove over low heat, or purchase a special heating unit designed especially for paraffin baths. Either way, use caution to avoid being burned by a too hot mixture.

"Allow plenty of time for rest in between concentrated work hours. Know your limits and be assertive in not exceeding them."

"I exercise and stretch my whole body in the mornings. I try to release the tension building in my neck or back during each break."

"I put an ice pack on my elbow every chance I get. It really helps!"

CORTISONE

Cortisone (a type of **steroid**—a strong anti-inflammatory medication) injections may be recommended by your physician at this stage, usually giving temporary relief. 80% of patients will feel an improvement in pain and numbness; however, one year later only 20% of those patients will remain pain-free. Like other anti-inflammatory medications, cortisone injections should be viewed as a *temporary* measure to relieve acute symptoms, not as cure. Long term usage of cortisone can do more harm than good; side effects include elevated blood pressure, menstrual disturbances, muscle weakness, and acne.

At this point, significant reduction (or even complete, temporary stoppage) of the aggravating activity is generally suggested. For many people, this option is difficult to accept.

"I depend on my hands for my work. If I stopped using my hands, how would I make a living?"

"For a while, I gave up every activity involving the use of my hands: writing, tennis, sewing. It was a difficult way to live!"

Depending on the amount of nerve damage, the success of the treatment program, and the patient's ability to make changes in habits and lifestyle, Stage II CTS patients can either achieve a full or partial recovery *or* the condition can worsen into Stage III Carpal Tunnel Syndrome.

6

STAGE
III

When patients have moderate to severe symptoms for more than one year or have consistent weakness and/or atrophy of muscles in the thumb, and electromyographic tests show significant abnormalities we call this **Stage III** Carpal Tunnel Syndrome.

At this point, there is significant damage to the median nerve and it is difficult to relieve symptoms with any kind of conservative treatment (ice, splints, massage). Patients in Stage III generally experience nearly constant pain in the wrist and hand, and/or numbness and tingling in the fingers. Grip strength can be affected, and the patient may have trouble picking up or holding things. When the thumb and index finger of the injured hand are pinched together, they can be separated easily due to weakness of the muscles. The muscle at the base of the thumb may actually begin to shrink in size. At this point, there is no question that some kind of medical intervention is necessary to prevent further, and possibly irreparable, nerve damage.

Orthopedic surgeons can fashion a device that goes beyond the immobilization of the wrist splint—a sort of removable cast that is worn everywhere except the shower or bath. In Stage III, it is advisable to completely discontinue any activity that will worsen the injury. The nerve needs a chance to heal, and it can't without rest.

SURGERY

If damage to the nerve has progressed to the point where more conservative methods fail, medical doctors will usually suggest surgery as soon as possible to release the entrapped nerve.

Under local or general anesthetic, the transverse ligament is cut and released, relieving the pressure on the median nerve. Recovery time varies depending on the degree of damage to the median nerve and the technique used by the surgeon. If you are asleep under general anesthetic during the surgery, you will need some time to recover from its effects as well. You will wake up with a large cast covering the hand and wrist, which will be removed in a week or two by your doctor and replaced with a lighter, gauze bandage. The scar from this type of surgery is barely noticeable in most cases.

Physicians fear that the longer the nerves are involved and irritated, the less the chances for successful surgery. If you are diagnosed in this stage of CTS, discuss your options with your doctor. Is surgery necessary, or could a more conservative course of treatment be attempted first without risk of further damage to the nerve? If surgery is recommended, the patient should ask questions, perhaps even seek a second opinion before making a final decision. As with any medical procedure, a successful result cannot be guaranteed. Surgery to release the transverse ligament can fail for a variety of reasons. The nerve may have been irreparably damaged prior to surgery or scar tissue from the surgery itself could create more pressure on the nerve. Talk to your doctor about your particular case. S/he will be able to examine the results from your diagnostic tests and give you some idea of your chances for a successful recovery.

Shots, surgery, acupuncture, electrical stimulation, chiropractic ... these can all be effective in treating CTS in its varying stages. The right treatment varies from person to person. The best way to ensure a successful recovery is to learn all you can about your treatment options. Don't hesitate to ask your doctor or health practitioner about anything that's on your mind.

"My surgery went very well and I noticed a huge improvement right away. After a month off to recover, though, I went back to work and within a year had developed CTS again. I didn't really get well until I modified my work habits, posture, and diet."

"When I woke up from the surgery, I immediately noticed that the feeling in my fingers had returned. Recovery was easy—I'd been in so much pain before the operation I barely felt discomfort from the stitches and the incision."

"Even though I had bilateral surgeries, I still have tingling fingertips at times but no 'asleep hands.' When I adjust my posture, the tingling goes away soon after."

7

PREVENTION

When working with new employees on proper job habits and injury prevention, the first thing we stress is this: *you don't have to get it!* Carpal Tunnel Syndrome is not an inevitable part of using your hands a lot. However, it does require effort and commitment on your part to ensure healthy arms and hands, and that's what this chapter is about. Just like a dancer or a professional athlete, you must prepare your body to perform with minimal risk of injury.

Until recently, many people were unaware of what this syndrome is called. They may have attributed their symptoms to overwork, stress, tension, or assumed it was a natural part of their particular profession. Unfortunately, not all physicians are familiar enough with overuse injuries to be able to identify the cause and appropriate treatment. Patients have been told to put up with it, to stop what they were doing, or to wait until it became worse. Often the patient's condition would deteriorate to the point where conservative treatment programs were no longer effective, and complete immobilization of the hands and arms and/or surgery were the only alternatives.

This chapter is especially addressed to those of you with mild or no symptoms. If you are working in a field with a high incidence of Carpal Tunnel Syndrome (hairdressers, computer operators, typists, assembly workers, foodservers, musicians, butchers, sign language interpreters—any occupation that requires repetitive or awkward motion of the hands or arms), there are steps you can take *now* to prevent the symptoms from occurring or worsening. And if you are in the moderate to severe stages of CTS, it's not too late to learn some new techniques for warming up, stretching, and improving your posture to prevent further damage and relieve the pain or numbness you may be experiencing.

SELF-TESTING

You can check your own arms and hands to see if any problems are developing. The aforementioned Phalen's and Tinel's tests can be done regularly at home. [See Chapter 3, Figs. 13 and 14.] You can also check points along the elbow [Fig. 21], on the outside and inside of the arm, for pain and swelling. Tenderness in these

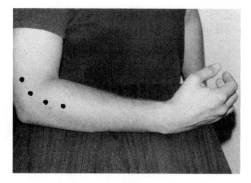 areas suggests that the muscles in the arms may be working excessively.

Stiffness, tightness, pain and/or restricted movement from the neck down into the upper shoulders or arms can be a warning that the arms and hands may eventually develop some problems.

Figure 21. Sore points along the elbow

These muscles should be treated using methods described in Chapters 4 and 5 and the joints in the neck examined to ensure maximum mobility and reduce the stiffness and pain.

WRIST SHAPE
AND CARPAL TUNNEL SYNDROME

A three year study at Ohio State University found three times greater evidence of nerve damage in autoworkers with "square" wrists as compared to those with "rectangular" ones. A "square" wrist was defined as one that was almost as thick as it was wide. The doctors involved in the study speculated that the way tendons lay in the "square" wrist may cause greater pressure on the nerve. Using a caliper from a medical or art supply store, measure both the height and width at the crease closest to the palm. Divide the thickness measurement by the width. A ratio of 0.7 or higher indicates a "square" wrist and possible increased risk for CTS.

EXERCISES FOR THE HAND

Overuse can leave the muscles of the hand feeling stiff, weak, or sore. There may be a lack of grip strength, or problems with coordination, especially with small, intricate tasks. Massage, moist heat, paraffin baths are all effective in relieving some of these symptoms, but you should also begin to strengthen the hand to achieve full rehabilitation. As with all exercises in this book, if there is significant pain present, do not attempt these exercises without consulting your health-care practitioner first.

A simple stretch for the hand starts with the palm flat down on a table. Arch the hand by pressing down with the thumb and little finger. Count to five, the release. Repeat 10–15 times, two or three times a day. Some CTS patients have gotten good results from exercising the hand using a special kind of therapy putty. We like the Rhino Gripper™ [see Appendix C], an inexpensive foam device contoured for the hand which can be used in numerous ways to tone and strengthen key muscle groups in the hands and forearms.

STRENGTHENING THE ARMS

It is important to build up the muscles in the arms and upper body as well to allow the muscles to function as fully as possible and

Figure 22.

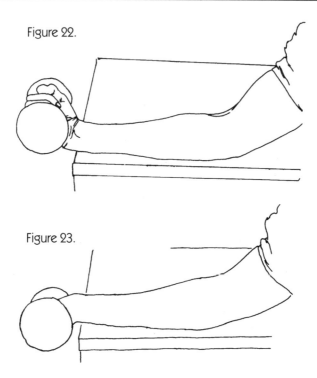

Figure 23.

to divert pressure off the vulnerable areas of the wrist. These exercises are effective *as long as the arm is not painful.* If you are experiencing pain, continue with ice and a forearm or wrist brace until you can put pressure on the arm without pain.

These exercises are done with the arm straight out and supported. Rest your arm on a table, arm of a chair, etc., holding a 1–2 pound weight in the hand, with the palm up. The hand is then *slightly* raised, the movement repeated ten times, then relaxed [Fig. 22]. Turn the arm over (palm down), and lower the hand *slightly* ten times [Fig. 23]. If you watch the arms while performing these exercises, you will see the muscles near the elbow working as you flex and extend. **Please note**: do not hyperextend or hyperflex the wrist with this exercise. Not only will the wrong muscles be used, but it can exaggerate the very problem you are trying to alleviate. Only a slight movement is needed, no more than an inch or two. Arm strengthening exercises should only be done when there is no pain or inflammation present when examining your elbow. If you feel discomfort, place a forearm brace on the arm *below* where it hurts, and apply ice to the injured part of the elbow on a daily basis until the inflammation subsides. If any pain is felt during or after the exercises, talk with your health-care practitioner before trying again.

On the other hand, if these movements feel too restrained and you are ready for something more, you can begin a program of strengthening not only your arms, but your chest and upper back muscles, too. Strengthening your upper body will take some of the strain off the hand and arm muscles that you use so often. A program with weights, exercise bands, and/or isometrics, approved by your health-care practitioner, can help you to not only recover but increase your strength and muscle tone, possibly preventing any further problems from occuring.

WARM-UP EXERCISES

Can you imagine a professional dancer taking the stage without warming up first? Never! Nor should *you* attempt any activity that taxes your hands and arms without stretching and warming up your muscles first.

Warm-up exercises relieve tension and relax muscles. It is much harder to injure a loose, relaxed muscle than a tight, tense one. Here are some exercises [Figs. 24–33] designed to warm up your hands, arms, shoulders, and neck. Practice them every morning before you start your day, during breaks, and at the end of the day to "cool down." They are best done while in a sitting position, feet flat on the floor.

 Do not continue any movement that feels painful.

Figure 24–Wrist Stretch
Place palms together in front of chest, fingers pointed up. Keeping palms together, slowly raise elbows upward as far as possible, pressing fingers together in backward direction.

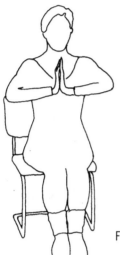

Figure 24

Figure 25–Shoulder Shrug
Slowly shrug shoulders as high as you can, hold for a count of five, then release. Repeat five times.

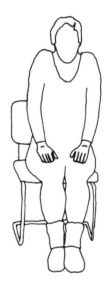

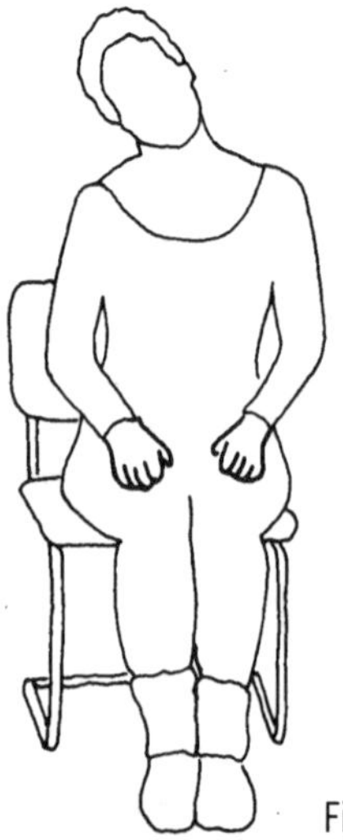

Figure 25

Figure 26–Neck Rotation
Allow the head to drop forward, then move it slowly in a full circle to the right. Repeat to opposite side. Next, starting with the neck as straight as possible, slowly tilt the head down toward right shoulder, hold for a count of five, then come back up to original position. Repeat to the left, back and front positions.

Figure 26

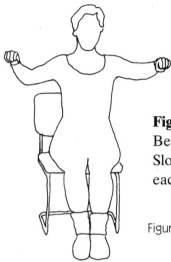

Figure 27 – Chest Expansion Stretch
Bend arms and raise to shoulder height. Slowly pull arms backward, elbows toward each other behind back.

Figure 27

Figure 28 – Upper Back Stretch
Place left hand on right shoulder. Hold left arm right above elbow with the right hand. Slowly pull left elbow, stretching toward right shoulder. Repeat for opposite side.

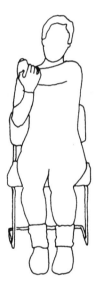

Figure 28

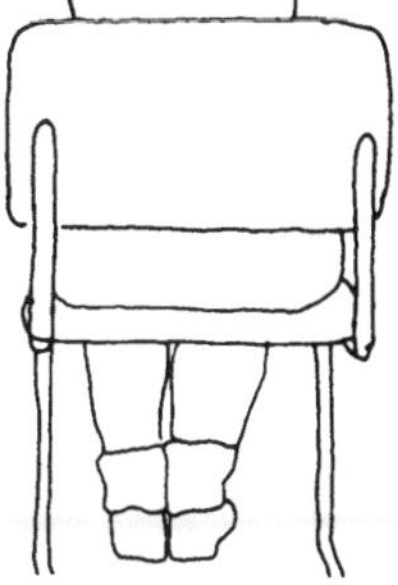

Figure 29 – Shoulder Stretch
Bring right hand behind head to upper back. Gently pull right elbow back and downward with left hand, moving the right hand down toward the center of the upper back. Repeat on opposite side.

Figure 29

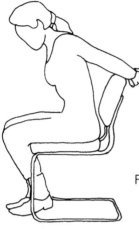

Figure 30–Shoulder Rotation
Clasp hands behind back. With arms extended straight, slowly lift arms upward.

Figure 30

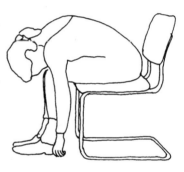

Figure 31–Back Stretch
Bend forward as far as you can, dropping head, shoulders and arms forward.

Figure 31

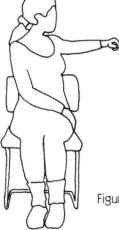

Figure 32–Upper Body Rotation
Grasp left hip with right hand. Bend left arm and raise to shoulder height. Rotate upper body to left while pulling on hip with right hand. Repeat for opposite side.

Figure 32

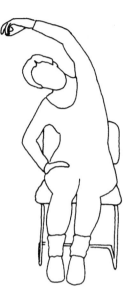

Figure 33 – Side Rotation
Place right hand on hip (careful not to hyperextend the wrist). With left arm extended over head, slowly stretch upper body to right. Repeat for opposite side.

Figure 33

EXERCISES FOR THE NECK

Anyone who uses his/her hands and arms frequently will also need to be aware of the neck's involvement in the development of overuse injuries. The neck must be kept as mobile and flexible as possible to ensure that there is little or no pressure on the nerve roots coming out of the cervical spine. Reducing pressure in the cervical spine optimizes the functioning of the nerves going down into the arm.

Simple mobility exercises are necessary to keep the neck flexible. These exercises [Figs. 34–38] should be done as often as possible, at least three times a day. We recommend one of the sessions per day be performed while standing under a comfortably hot shower.

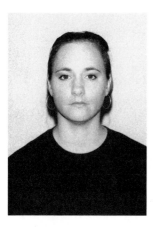

Figure 34–Sit in a normal position with the head facing straight ahead.

Figure 34

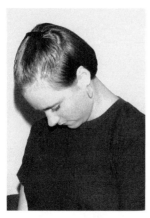

Figure 35–Nod the head forward, touching the chin to the chest three times. After each nod, return to a normal position of looking straight ahead.

Figure 35

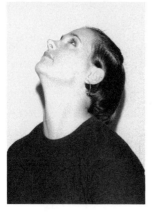

Figure 36–Tilt the head back as far as is comfortable. This should be a smooth backward motion, not in a jerking manner. Do this three times.

Figure 36

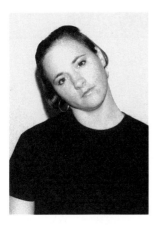

Figure 37–While facing forward, tilt the head to the right so that the right ear touches the right shoulder. This is done three times. Keep looking forward and do not rotate the head, but instead laterally flex the head as much and as painlessly as possible. Do the same with the left side.

Figure 37

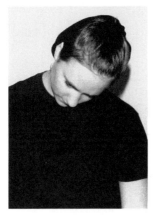

Figure 38–Roll the head around (circumduct) counter-clockwise, three times, smoothly and without jerking motions, in as wide a range of motion as is painlessly possible.

Last of all, roll the head around clockwise as described above.

Figure 38

These exercises should feel comfortable. Again, do *not* attempt any exercise if pain is present before, during, or after you've finished. Care should be taken to stretch only within a comfortable range—more is not necessarily better.

ACUPRESSURE AND MASSAGE

There are acupressure points along the neck, middle back and shoulder area that can help relieve tense muscles, thereby allowing the arm muscles to function better, as well as enhancing the nerve supply to the arm.

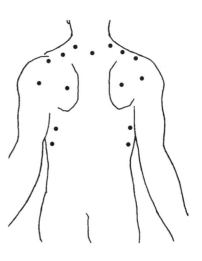

Figure 39 shows the points to work on. Apply gentle pressure with the thumb or finger directly to the points. You may feel a small knot or nodule. Ask the person to breathe deeply and slowly three times while you

Figure 39. Acupressure points

apply a constant low level of pressure downward (not too hard!). Be careful of the points along the top of the shoulders, as they are typically fairly tender.

There are a variety of books, tapes, and classes available on the art of massage. We strongly encourage anyone involved in an activity that creates tension, tightness, and restriction across the neck and upper back to take the time to learn some techniques of massage. Check into your local adult education or community college district to see if massage classes are offered.

8

—ERGONOMICS—
CREATING A HEALTHY
WORK ENVIRONMENT

Observe an injured worker on the job, and chances are you'll spot a problem with posture and/or the physical layout of the work station. With some retraining and simple improvements in the workplace, injuries can be decreased and even prevented.

—ERGONOMICS—
A NEW IDEA IN OFFICE DESIGN

Ergonomics is a big word for a simple concept; basically, it refers to the idea of creating a work environment that promotes physical health and comfort while optimizing job performance. Overuse injuries are at epidemic levels in the workplace. Employers are discovering that it is actually more cost effective to make the initial investment in furniture and equipment designed to prevent physical stress than to deal with the problem of work-related injuries down the line. Because of the rise in CTS and overuse injuries, office and computer supply stores offer an abundant selection of chairs, desks, wrist rests, document holders, monitor stands, and other devices designed to minimize risk of injury.

THE RIGHT CHAIR

Many injuries start with poorly designed seating. An uncomfortable chair leads to postural problems, which in turn throw off the alignment of the spine and impair nerve function to the arms and hands. So, let's start with chair design. The ideal chair should be adjustable to a height that is comfortable for you—16 to 20 inches from the floor is best. Your weight should be forward and your arms at desk height. Both feet should rest flat on the floor; if they don't reach, use a footrest. Hips and knees should be at the same height to reduce stress on the legs. The lower back needs support, whether by the chair itself or through the use of a cushion or rolled-up towel.

Even the best chair won't help if you slump or slouch. Keep your spine and head upright, and prevent slouching by sitting *back* into the chair.

THE COMPUTERIZED OFFICE

Spending long hours at a computer can take its toll on your hands, wrists, and neck, leading to strain and injury. However, there are many things you can do to improve your workstation and create a more comfortable environment.

First, raise your computer monitor to *eye level* to reduce strain on the neck. If you are bending your head down to see the screen comfortably, you are putting excess strain on the cervical spine. There are a variety of monitor stands available in any computer supply store, or you can simply place your monitor on a stack of phone books. The same principle applies when working with documents. Do not crane or bend your neck to read the copy. Use a document holder to keep your papers at eye level and take pressure off your neck as you work.

Keep hands and wrists in a comfortable, relaxed position— not too high or held at an awkward angle. Forearms should be at right angles to the body, with the forearm parallel to the floor. Seventy to ninety degrees is the ideal angle for typing or data entry tasks.

The use of a wrist rest is mandatory if you spend much time at a keyboard. An excellent wrist rest to try is the Wrist Reminder™ by MicroComputer Accessories, Inc. Designed specifically to prevent or alleviate symptoms of overuse injuries, the Wrist Reminder is a comfortable wrist band with a plastic palm support, which provides support and limits wrist flexion while still allowing full range of motion of the fingers. Microcomputer Accessories is a leader in ergonomically-designed wrist support products, including keyboard platforms, adjustable wrist rests, and the Wrist Trolley™—gliding pads that attach to your keyboard. See Appendix C for information on these products. An idea you can try yourself is just to place a small, folded towel at the base of your keyboard. Even a little extra support can go a long way in alleviating fatigue and tension.

You may need to do some rearranging of your work station to achieve a setup that allows you to perform your duties *and* prevent injuries. Check your local computer or office supply store to ask about monitor stands, wrist rests, document holders, and other ideas to prevent repetitive motion injuries. There is even software available that, once installed in your computer, will remind you at set intervals to stretch or take a break!

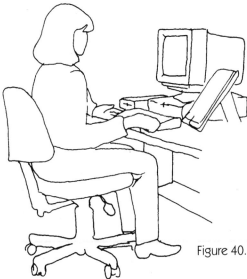

Figure 40. A well-designed work station

WRITING BY HAND

If you write a lot by hand, purchase a few inexpensive pen/pencil grips to ease the strain on your fingers. Grips can also be used on paint brushes, crochet hooks and knitting needles, drafting tools, even toothbrushes, and come in a variety of sizes and styles (see Appendix for ordering information). Most patients we interviewed reported that writing or drawing by hand for a prolonged period nearly always worsened symptoms considerably. Be sure to take frequent breaks to relax the hand and arm muscles if you are doing a lot of writing.

STANDING

Many of the same principles apply to those of you who work in a standing position. Keeping your spine in an aligned position [Fig. 41] helps to alleviate strain.

Imagine a string running through the top of your head, down your back to your hips, holding your head erect and spine straight. The shoulders should be back, and take care not to allow the hips to rotate out and back. Figure 42 illustrates a posture that is incorrect and may well lead to injuries.

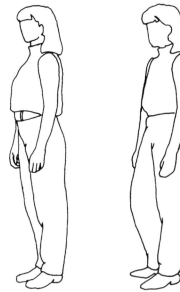

Figure 41. Correct   Figure 42. Incorrect

9

STRESS MANAGEMENT

By now you are beginning to see that attitude plays a large part in your overall health. Everyone experiences stress, but why do some people seem to be able to sail through life while others of us become burned out, fatigued, and even succumb to illness as a result of stress?

There is no question that a person living with chronic pain may go through stages of fear, depression, and anger. They may be told the symptoms are "all in their head" or "psychosomatic." Impairment of the use of the hands is devastating, and people suffering from Carpal Tunnel Syndrome often report feelings of helplessness and isolation. Remember, until recently very little information was available about CTS.

Just as you have learned that physical wellness can only be achieved when you make the time to meet your body's needs, maintaining emotional health requires the same attention. And, like the stretching exercises and self-help techniques you have learned to relieve your physical symptoms, there are many ways to alleviate stress.

Try the techniques listed in this chapter. When you find one that works for you, set aside a special time every day to practice in a quiet place. Even if you can only spare ten minutes out of your hectic schedule, it is important to schedule a time devoted entirely to taking care of yourself. The best time is early in the morning when you are rested. Set the clock fifteen minutes earlier if necessary. Before bed is another good time to unwind by yourself.

RELAXATION EXERCISE

This exercise in progressive relaxation is designed to help you train yourself to feel the difference between relaxation and tension. By understanding what being completely relaxed feels like, you will more easily notice when your muscles are beginning to tighten up in response to stress or fatigue. People who are in pain tend to keep their muscles tense all the time, almost as if they were protecting the injured limb.

Try reading the following exercise into a tape recorder so that you can practice without referring back to the book. Sit comfortably, in loose clothing, and remember to take slow, deep breaths throughout the exercise.

Start by focusing your attention on your toes. Clench your toes as tight as you can, and hold for a count of ten. Slowly release the muscles until they are completely relaxed.

Next, flex your feet by pointing your toes up and back. You will feel a tightening in your calf muscles. Hold for a count of ten, then slowly release.

Tighten the muscles of your buttocks, thighs, and stomach. Feel your legs lift slightly as you count to ten. Slowly release. Continue taking slow, deep breaths as you relax. As you visualize filling your lungs with clean, pure air, see any tension leaving your body each time you exhale.

Next, you will tense the muscles of your upper body. Clench your fists, arms straight out at your sides. Tighten your arms and chest muscles. Hold as you count to ten, then release.

Next, tighten your neck. Push your head back and clench your jaw, lips tight together. Hold for a count of ten, then release slowly.

Remember to keep breathing, slowly and deeply.

Last, tense the muscles of your face. Open your mouth as wide as you can, as if you are yawning. Tighten your eyes by squeezing them shut as tightly as you can. Frown and wrinkle your nose. Hold the muscles tight for a count of ten. Let the tension go as you gently relax.

POSITIVE MENTAL IMAGING

There is growing evidence that our thoughts have a powerful influence on our health. Certainly it is true that holding a calm, pleasant image in the mind can lower heart rate and blood pressure. A visualization to help heal an injured arm might go like this:

First, find a comfortable place where you can totally relax without interruption. You can put on a tape of soothing music, or tape this exercise and play it back. We will focus this exercise on the right arm, but you can adapt this exercise to any part of the body.

Imagine your right arm feeling warm and heavy. Feel the blood moving through the shoulder, elbow, forearm, wrist, hand, and fingers. Your fingers feel warm and relaxed. Now, starting at your shoulder, imagine a ball of white light glowing its way down your arm. The light moves slowly, stopping at any sore spots to melt away the pain.

See the light moving down your upper arm, elbow, forearm, wrist, hand, and fingers. Hold the glowing white ball in your hand for a moment, then let it go, imagining that it is carrying away all the soreness and tension. Feel your arm become light and weightless.

MEDITATION

Meditation is a powerful tool for quieting the mind and reducing stress. There are probably hundreds of different techniques for meditation, so you may need to do some research to find one that feels right for you. Here is one you can try:

Find a quiet place where you can be alone and undisturbed for 15–30 minutes. Sit in a comfortable position, cross-legged if you can without strain, spine straight. Lie down if that feels better. You can keep your eyes open slightly or close them. Begin by taking slow, deep, even breaths. Again, visualize all tension and stress leaving your body each time you exhale. Clear your mind of all thoughts. Some people find it helpful to chant a **mantra**: a word or phrase repeated during the meditation that can keep you focused. Try saying "Om" with each exhale, stretching the word until you are ready to take your next breath. At first it may be difficult to concentrate. If your mind wanders and you find unwanted thoughts popping up, just observe the thoughts and let them go. Don't get caught up in your thoughts: keep breathing and stay focused.

AFFIRMATIONS

In order to effect positive changes in our lives, we must replace our old, self-defeating tapes with new, empowering messages. Affirmations are a way to "reprogram" your thoughts and break down old defenses that create stress and illness. Working with one or two statements at a time, write the affirmation down in a journal (some examples are listed below). Next to it, write the immediate response you feel about the idea. Your response to an affirmation like "I enjoy perfect health" may be "No way!!" That's fine. Keep writing. Notice the ways your responses change as you begin to assimilate the positive messages. When you feel ready to move on to new ones, feel free to change. You'll be able to come up with your own affirmations that work best for you. Stick with positive messages. For example, "I don't hate my job" would be better phrased as "I enjoy and feel fulfilled by my work." Affirmations can also be read into a tape recorder; you can purchase a continuous loop cassette tape (the kind used for answering machines) and incorporate affirmations into your relaxation or meditation routines.

- I listen with love to my body's messages.
- I am at peace with myself and others.
- I love and approve of myself.
- I joyously flow with life and each new experience.
- I enjoy perfect health.

- I receive the love and support I need.
- I am willing to change.
- I am responsible for myself.
- I recognize and take care of my own needs.
- Everyone is responsible for their own behavior and choices.
- My needs are as important as everyone else's.

BIOFEEDBACK

Biofeedback involves the use of a special machine that, when its sensors are attached to points on the body, can monitor heart rate, temperature, brain wave activity, and muscle tension. Once you are "hooked up" to the machine, it is easy to follow your body's reactions by looking at a digital readout or listening for audio tones that speed up or slow down. You can then begin to identify thought patterns that effect your heart rate, muscle tension, etc., and train yourself to relax and influence the readings from the machine. Home biofeedback units are available, but formal training is necessary to get a thorough understanding of the techniques involved. Your best bet is a trained professional, at least to get you started on the right foot.

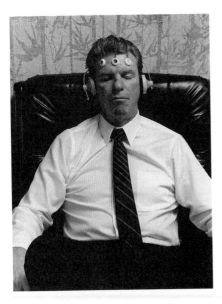

Figure 43. Biofeedback

10

YOUR RIGHTS AND RESPONSIBILITIES

We hope this book has led you to think of yourself as an *active* participant in your own treatment and recovery process. That attitude shift is essential to a successful treatment program. Our society tends to view doctors as omnipotent and Godlike, while patients are passive, trusting, and uninformed. It is in your best interest to become informed about *any* injury or illness you experience. Don't be afraid to ask questions, read, or talk to others with the same symptoms. Knowledge is your best tool in maintaining your health.

CHOOSING THE RIGHT DOCTOR

Traditionally, people choose a particular physician by a referral from someone they know. Doctors may also refer patients to another physician or specialist for a specific problem. Patients may not be aware that, although referrals are generally made with the best intentions, your doctor may be giving you the name of an acquaintance, former classmate, or fellow club member: not necessarily the best choice for your particular needs. You may hear that a certain doctor is the very best in the state, country, or even world, and s/he may indeed be technically proficient. But when choosing a physician, technical proficiency is not enough. Is the doctor empathetic, compassionate, and patient enough to allow an injured person to follow a less than traditional program? Is s/he aware and up-to-date about the newest and most innovative methods of treatment?

Not all doctors or health professionals are familiar with accumulative trauma-type injuries. Sometimes, if the symptoms are not considered severe enough, treatment will be delayed. When choosing a physician, ask the following questions:

- What kind of experience do you have treating accumulative trauma injuries?
- What kinds of cases have you treated and what were the results?
- Do you refer many of your patients out for surgery? Physical therapy?
- What is your criteria for change or stoppage of treatment?
- What do you consider to be the results of successful treatment?

The doctor should be willing to discuss these questions and listen to your considerations as well.

Physicians have many different philosophies and ways of looking at patients with pain. You may want to consider the objectivity of health-care practitioners who are employed by industries or insurance companies. Is a large percentage of the physician's practice derived from those companies? It is doubtful that a physician would jeopardize a patient's health unnecessarily; however, there may be a slant to his or her philosophy, particularly when the injury is work-related.

Perhaps a better way of locating a doctor is to ask family, friends, or co-workers for referrals. If overuse injuries are prevalent in your field, ask others who have had similar problems about their experiences, good or bad reactions, successes and failures in treatment, etc. Word of mouth, especially from people you trust, is an excellent way to find a doctor you feel good about. And that, above all else, should be your main criteria when selecting a health-care practitioner. You should feel comfortable enough with your doctor to ask questions and have them answered simply and politely, without feeling patronized or rushed. After all, in a sense the doctor is the employee of the patient. You are paying for a service; the doctor is working for *you*.

GETTING A SECOND OPINION

Obtaining a second opinion may be a good idea, especially if for any reason you don't feel completely comfortable with your doctor. Get the name of another doctor in the same type of specialty; if you saw a chiropractor, see another chiropractor. If you talked to an orthopedist, see another orthopedist. For the most objective evaluation, find the new doctor on your own rather than asking for a referral from your first physician. Let both doctors make an objective diagnosis about your condition and recommendations for treatment.

After they've given their opinions, feel free to share what the other doctor said and ask for an explanation of any differences in opinion. Don't be afraid to ask questions; your doctor should not become defensive or angry when asked to explain his or her criteria (if they do, you may want to look elsewhere for your health care).

Once you get the collective opinion of one specialty of health-care practitioners (M.D., chiropractor, osteopath, acupuncturist, etc.), you can also inquire into a different type of care. Don't be alarmed if you find there are disagreements between the different specialties. A medical doctor may or may not be supportive of the care you receive from an acupuncturist, or vice versa. There is something of value to be learned from a variety of health-care practitioners, in whatever specialty they practice. Often, patients find the most effective treatment involves a *combination* of techniques: traditional medical care with massage, chiropractic with homeopathy, etc. Look for a primary-care health professional who is open-minded enough to discuss any and all ideas you have about treatment. It is your job to determine what works best for you, and it is *important* to explore all your options; the treatment you ultimately choose affects your future and quality of life, and is worth the extra trouble.

A ONE-MONTH TRIAL FOR MILD SYMPTOMS

If EMG testing is negative, it is safe to say there is probably not significant damage to the median nerve yet. A one-month trial on a conservative treatment program should not jeopardize the nerve or cause irreversible damage. You and your physician can decide on some specific goals, outline a treatment plan, then retest in one month to see if there are any changes. If your symptoms improve, great! Continue treatment until symptoms are gone, then begin a strengthening and stretching program to rehabilitate the arm.

If your symptoms plateau for four to six weeks, discuss ways to address the remaining symptoms with your doctor. If treatment brings no improvement, it may be time to try something less conservative.

YOUR RESPONSIBILITIES

Even the best doctor in the world cannot help you if you don't commit 100% to following the recommended treatment program. Stretching, warm-up exercises, icing painful spots, and/or lifestyle changes are *your* responsibility. Often patients go to a doctor expecting to be made well, given a magic pill that will heal them in a day or so. Carpal Tunnel Syndrome and overuse injuries don't happen overnight, nor will they disappear in an instant. Anti-inflammatory medication or a shot of cortisone can bring quick relief, but the injury is virtually guaranteed to progressively worsen if changes in work and personal habits aren't made. It is vital that you see yourself and your physician as a team, both actively working toward the same goal.

Many occupations require repetitive movements that can lead to injury. It is time to rethink old attitudes about what employees are physically capable of doing, and combine the desire to perform our jobs well and to the best of our ability with a respect for our physical well-being.

KEEPING A JOURNAL

It is helpful for both you and your doctor if you keep track of your symptoms on a daily basis, including which activities make you feel better or worse. Habits, work duties, diet, exercise, menstruation—all can have a great deal of influence on your symptoms.

Keeping a daily journal can help you see patterns developing, and whether you are improving or going downhill. Day to day changes can seem slow, even going backwards at times, so a journal kept over a long period can show slow but steady changes.

Start out by assigning a numerical value from 0 to 10 to the pain levels in your hands, wrists, arms, neck, and/or back. (If you are experiencing numbness, tingling, weakness, etc., record those levels, too.) Use 10 to indicate the very worst pain, and 0 as completely pain-free.

Improvements can be noted by a decrease in the numbers or the fact that it begins to take longer before symptoms arise. For example, suppose your wrist initially began to hurt at a level of 7 after ten minutes of typing. After two weeks of treatment it may still hurt, but now it takes 30 minutes before you are at the same level of 7.

Overuse injuries are not only caused by repetitive motion at work. Many people engage in hobbies that involve the hands: crafts, drawing, sewing, carpentry, knitting, operating a computer, or sporting activities. It is important to note whether your hands are being overused, hyperextended or hyperflexed in these non-work related activities as well, and apply what you've learned to the activities of your everyday life.

Keep a record of how your diet affects your symptoms. Do you notice an increase in pain and numbness after a meal high in salt? Do you feel sluggish a few hours after eating a candy bar? Do vitamin B supplements help?

In Appendix B we have provided a sample weekly chart to assist you in keeping track of your treatment and symptoms. Feel free to make copies or revise it in any way that works best for you.

WHO PAYS?
WORKER'S COMPENSATION
AND PRIVATE INSURANCE

With few exceptions, nearly every employee is covered by Worker's Compensation when injured on the job. The first step is to promptly report any injury to your immediate supervisor. You will be asked to complete a claim form describing the injury. In many states you are required initially to see the doctor who represents your employer's Worker's Compensation insurance company, then, after a specified time (usually 30 days), you can choose the health-care provider of your choice. The choice of health-care provider is even more significant when Worker's Compensation is involved; typically, these insurance companies discourage changing doctors more than once or twice, and only with an excellent reason.

Most injuries that occur on the job are caused by accidents, like a cut finger or a fall. Accumulative trauma is somewhat more complicated; it may be hard to pinpoint the exact date of injury, for example, if you are required to provide that information on a claim form.

Worker's Compensation can reimburse you for medical costs, lost wages, permanent disability, rehabilitation services, and even vocational training to prepare you for a different occupation. Benefits can vary depending on where you live. For information on Workers' Compensation in your state, call the nearest office of the State Division of Worker's Compensation. They can help you understand your rights and answer any questions you have. If you belong to a union, your representative should be able to advise you, as well. And, if none of these avenues are satisfactory, there are attorneys who specialize in Workers' Compensation law and can handle your claim for you.

If the injury interferes with your work but is not work-related (directly caused by the duties of your job), you may be eligible for some kind of state disability if you need time off to recover. Check with your employer's benefits office. If your injury is not work-related, your private medical insurance may cover some of the costs of medical treatment. Many insurance companies will now also cover chiropractic care and acupuncture. Check your policy to find out what services are covered.

Worker's Compensation can be an expensive solution for your employer and his/her insurance carrier. If several of your coworkers are experiencing problems similar to yours, it may be time to sit down and make some changes, whether in each worker's work station, in the scheduling of each shift, or in establishing a program to educate workers who are at risk. Often these kinds of changes cost much less in the long run than absences, surgeries, vocational rehabilitation, and retraining new personnel.

YOU ARE WORTH IT

The permanent, crippling effects of CTS can be devastating. The level of pain and discomfort can create the need for constant medication and severe limitations in lifestyle. People who suffer from chronic pain experience increased stress, side effects from accumulated levels of medication, and higher levels of drug and alcohol abuse and domestic problems. We have seen firsthand how these injuries affect lives, not only in terms of physical discomfort but in a constant stream of little things patients used to take for granted: opening a jar, sewing a button, shaking hands, doing push-ups, carrying a bag of groceries, writing a letter, chopping vegetables, and on and on. One of the saddest comments shared by a CTS patient when describing the worst thing about having the injury was "When I walk along the beach with my daughter, I can't feel her hand in mine anymore."

Many of these injuries can be prevented, and many of those already experiencing symptoms can find relief. We strongly encourage you to become an active participant in your treatment. Read, ask questions, and experiment with what you learn. Follow your health-care practitioner's advice, and keep your eyes and ears open to new ideas, techniques, and therapies. Apply as much of the information you've learned from this book as possible. Changes in work habits, lifestyle, diet, and attitude can not only help you recover from Carpal Tunnel Syndrome, but will also vastly improve the quality of your life. Make taking care of yourself a **priority**: *you are worth it.*

APPENDIX A
OVERUSE INJURY CHECK LIST

Use this check list to keep a record of your symptoms. It can also be helpful to share with your physician when you go for an examination. Make copies of this page to document your progress as you go through treatment.

1. PAIN: 0=no pain, 10=worst pain

    Fingers   L ____   R ____

    (which fingers?   _____)

    Hand   L ____   R ____

    Wrist   L ____   R ____

    Forearm   L ____   R ____

    Shoulder   L ____   R ____

    Shoulder Blade   L ____   R ____

    Neck   L ____   R ____

2. NUMBNESS: 1=never, 2=occasionally, 3=most of the time, 4=constant

    Fingers   L ____   R ____

    (which fingers?   _____)

    Hand   L ____   R ____

    Wrist   L ____   R ____

    Forearm   L ____   R ____

    Shoulder   L ____   R ____

    Shoulder Blade   L ____   R ____

    Neck   L ____   R ____

3. TINGLING: 1=never, 2=occasionally, 3=most of the time, 4=constant

Fingers   L ____   R ____

(which fingers?   _____)

Hand   L ____   R ____

Wrist   L ____   R ____

Forearm   L ____   R ____

Shoulder   L ____   R ____

Shoulder Blade   L ____   R ____

Neck   L ____   R ____

4. WEAKNESS: 1=never, 2=occasionally, 3=most of the time, 4=constant

Fingers   L ____   R ____

(which fingers?   _____)

Hand   L ____   R ____

Wrist   L ____   R ____

Forearm   L ____   R ____

Shoulder   L ____   R ____

Shoulder Blade   L ____   R ____

Neck   L ____   R ____

APPENDIX B
SAMPLE JOURNAL

Keeping a journal: Recording your daily habits and symptoms on a chart like this one will help you keep track of your progress as you go through your treatment plan. This is valuable information for your physician as well.

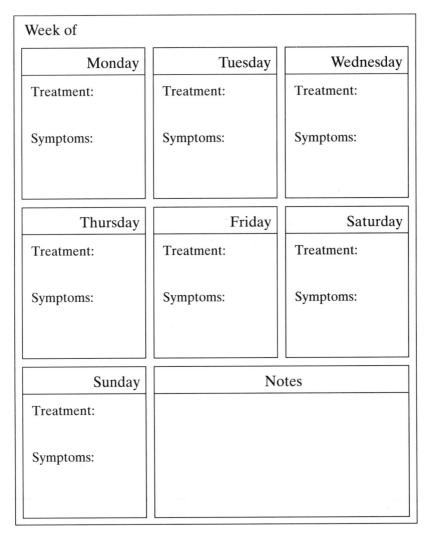

Week of

Monday	Tuesday	Wednesday
Treatment: Symptoms:	Treatment: Symptoms:	Treatment: Symptoms:

Thursday	Friday	Saturday
Treatment: Symptoms:	Treatment: Symptoms:	Treatment: Symptoms:

Sunday	Notes
Treatment: Symptoms:	

Treatment: list any medications, therapy (massage, manipulation, physical therapy), self-help (ice, rest, splints, Warm-up/stretching, stress reduction), changes in diet, etc.

Symptoms: on a scale of 1–10, with 10 being the worst pain and 1 the least, rate any symptoms you experience each day. Specify whether you feel pain, numbness, tingling, or weakness.

Make a special note on days you use your arms and hands alot, so you can see how extra activity affects your symptoms.

APPENDIX C
ORDERING INFORMATION

For your convenience, we have compiled a brief list of some of the products that have proven effective in treating Carpal Tunnel Syndrome and overuse injury symptoms, and the companies where these products can be ordered. Check your own local medical supply companies, stores that specialize in natural foods or nutrition, computer supply distributers, drug stores; there are products out there that can help you, but it may take a bit of effort to find them.

1. **Traumeel ointment and tablets**
   Biological Homeopathic Industries Inc.
   11600 Cochiti S.E.
   Albuquerque, NM 87123
   1-800-621-7644

2. **Pen/Pencil Grippers**
   Grab On Products
   100 N. Avery Street
   Walla Walla, WA 99362
   1-800-8GRABON

3. **Sonassage Sonic Pain Reliever**
   Conair Corporation
   150 Milford Road
   East Windsor, NJ 08520
   1-800-3-CONAIR

4. **Wrist splints, forearm braces, cervical pillows, and other orthopedic supplies**
   Anabolic Laboratories
   P.O. Box C19508
   17802 Gillette Avenue
   Irvine, CA 92713
   1-714-863-0340

5. **Rhino Grippers Hand Strengthening System**
   Therapy Skill Builders
   3830 E. Bellvue/P.O. Box 42050-Y
   Tucson, AZ 85733
   1-602-323-7500

6. **Wrist Reminder**
   Microcomputer Accessories
   5405 Jandy Place/P.O. Box 66991
   Los Angeles, CA 90066
   1-213-301-9400

INDEX

accumulative trauma, 5, 62, 66
acetaminophen, 28
acromegaly, 6
acupressure, 50
acupuncture, xii, 10, 14–15, 23, 36, 67
affirmations, 58
alternative medicine, 10
anti-inflammatory medication, 28, 33, 64
Applied Kinesiology, 23
arthritis, 6, 29
aspirin, 28

biofeedback, 59
birth control pills, 31

carpal tunnel, 1–2
cervical pillows, 29, 73
chair design, 52
chi, 14
chiropractic, xii, 10–14, 36, 63, 67
computer, 5, 23, 39, 51–53, 73
Computerized Tomography (CT or CAT scan), 23
cortisone, 33, 64
cumulative trauma disorder, 1

DeQuervain's disease, 7
diabetes mellitis, 5
diagnostic tests, 21, 31, 36
document holders, 51–53
dynamometer, 22–23

edema, 12, 16
electromyography (EMG), 24–25, 35, 64
electrotherapy, 16
endorphins, 14–15
ergonomics, 51–53
exercise, 14, 16, 19, 27, 32–33, 41–50, 55–57, 64–65

forearm brace, 26–27, 31, 43, 73
"funny bone," 3, 6

ginger compress, 32
"golfer's elbow," 7

holistic medicine, 10
Homeopathy, 10, 15, 18, 32, 63
hyperextension, 4–5, 42, 66
hyperflexion, 4–5, 42, 66
hypothyroidism, 5

ibuprofen, 28
ice packs, 27, 33
immobilization, 26, 35, 39
insurance, medical, 13, 15, 62, 66–67
interferential current therapy, 11, 16–17

journal, 58, 65, 71

kidney dialysis, 5

Magnetic Resonance Imaging (MRI), 23
manipulation, 11, 14, 23, 72
massage, 11, 13, 18, 25–28, 31–32, 35, 41, 50, 63, 72
median nerve percussion test, *see* Tinel's test
median nerve, xi, 1–2, 4–5, 21–24, 35–36, 64
meditation, 57–58
menopause, 5
mental imaging, 57
moist heat, 27, 41
monitor stands, 51–53
multiple myeloma, 6

natural medicine, 10
neurologist, 24